DATE	TIME	NUMBER OF PUSH-UPS
DATE	TIME	NUMBER OF PUSH-UPS

DATE	TIME	NUMBER OF PUSH-UPS

DATE	TIME	NUMBER OF PUSH-UPS

DATE	TIME	NUMBER OF PUSH-UPS
DATE	TIME	NUMBER OF PUSH-UPS

DATE	TIME	NUMBER OF PUSH-UPS

DATE	TIME	NUMBER OF PUSH-UPS

DATE	TIME	NUMBER OF PUSH-UPS

DATE	TIME	NUMBER OF PUSH-UPS

DATE	TIME	NUMBER OF PUSH-UPS

DATE	TIME	NUMBER OF PUSH-UPS

DATE	TIME	NUMBER OF PUSH-UPS

DATE	TIME	NUMBER OF PUSH-UPS

DATE	TIME	NUMBER OF PUSH-UPS
DATE	TIME	NUMBER OF PUSH-UPS

DATE	TIME	NUMBER OF PUSH-UPS

DATE	TIME	NUMBER OF PUSH-UPS

DATE	TIME	NUMBER OF PUSH-UPS

DATE	TIME	NUMBER OF PUSH-UPS
DATE	TIME	NUMBER OF PUSH-UPS

DATE	TIME	NUMBER OF PUSH-UPS
DATE	TIME	NUMBER OF PUSH-UPS

DATE	TIME	NUMBER OF PUSH-UPS

DATE	TIME	NUMBER OF PUSH-UPS
DATE	TIME	NUMBER OF PUSH-UPS

DATE	TIME	NUMBER OF PUSH-UPS
DATE	TIME	NUMBER OF PUSH-UPS

DATE	TIME	NUMBER OF PUSH-UPS
DATE	TIME	NUMBER OF PUSH-UPS

DATE	TIME	NUMBER OF PUSH-UPS

DATE	TIME	NUMBER OF PUSH-UPS

DATE	TIME	NUMBER OF PUSH-UPS

DATE	TIME	NUMBER OF PUSH-UPS
DATE	TIME	NUMBER OF PUSH-UPS

DATE	TIME	NUMBER OF PUSH-UPS

DATE	TIME	NUMBER OF PUSH-UPS

DATE	TIME	NUMBER OF PUSH-UPS

DATE	TIME	NUMBER OF PUSH-UPS

DATE	TIME	NUMBER OF PUSH-UPS

DATE	TIME	NUMBER OF PUSH-UPS
DATE	TIME	NUMBER OF PUSH-UPS

DATE	TIME	NUMBER OF PUSH-UPS

DATE	TIME	NUMBER OF PUSH-UPS

DATE	TIME	NUMBER OF PUSH-UPS

DATE	TIME	NUMBER OF PUSH-UPS

DATE	TIME	NUMBER OF PUSH-UPS

DATE	TIME	NUMBER OF PUSH-UPS

DATE	TIME	NUMBER OF PUSH-UPS

DATE	TIME	NUMBER OF PUSH-UPS

DATE	TIME	NUMBER OF PUSH-UPS

DATE	TIME	NUMBER OF PUSH-UPS
DATE	TIME	NUMBER OF PUSH-UPS

DATE	TIME	NUMBER OF PUSH-UPS

DATE	TIME	NUMBER OF PUSH-UPS

DATE	TIME	NUMBER OF PUSH-UPS

DATE	TIME	NUMBER OF PUSH-UPS

DATE	TIME	NUMBER OF PUSH-UPS

DATE	TIME	NUMBER OF PUSH-UPS

DATE	TIME	NUMBER OF PUSH-UPS

DATE	TIME	NUMBER OF PUSH-UPS
	DATE	TIME	NUMBER OF PUSH-UPS

DATE	TIME	NUMBER OF PUSH-UPS

DATE	TIME	NUMBER OF PUSH-UPS

DATE	TIME	NUMBER OF PUSH-UPS

DATE	TIME	NUMBER OF PUSH-UPS

DATE	TIME	NUMBER OF PUSH-UPS

DATE	TIME	NUMBER OF PUSH-UPS

DATE	TIME	NUMBER OF PUSH-UPS

DATE	TIME	NUMBER OF PUSH-UPS

DATE	TIME	NUMBER OF PUSH-UPS

DATE	TIME	NUMBER OF PUSH-UPS

DATE	TIME	NUMBER OF PUSH-UPS

DATE	TIME	NUMBER OF PUSH-UPS

DATE	TIME	NUMBER OF PUSH-UPS

DATE	TIME	NUMBER OF PUSH-UPS

DATE	TIME	NUMBER OF PUSH-UPS

DATE	TIME	NUMBER OF PUSH-UPS

DATE	TIME	NUMBER OF PUSH-UPS

DATE	TIME	NUMBER OF PUSH-UPS

DATE	TIME	NUMBER OF PUSH-UPS
DATE	TIME	NUMBER OF PUSH-UPS

DATE	TIME	NUMBER OF PUSH-UPS

DATE	TIME	NUMBER OF PUSH-UPS

DATE	TIME	NUMBER OF PUSH-UPS
DATE	TIME	NUMBER OF PUSH-UPS

DATE	TIME	NUMBER OF PUSH-UPS

DATE	TIME	NUMBER OF PUSH-UPS

DATE	TIME	NUMBER OF PUSH-UPS

DATE	TIME	NUMBER OF PUSH-UPS

DATE	TIME	NUMBER OF PUSH-UPS

DATE	TIME	NUMBER OF PUSH-UPS
DATE	TIME	NUMBER OF PUSH-UPS

DATE	TIME	NUMBER OF PUSH-UPS

DATE	TIME	NUMBER OF PUSH-UPS

DATE	TIME	NUMBER OF PUSH-UPS
DATE	TIME	NUMBER OF PUSH-UPS

DATE	TIME	NUMBER OF PUSH-UPS

DATE	TIME	NUMBER OF PUSH-UPS
DATE	TIME	NUMBER OF PUSH-UPS

DATE	TIME	NUMBER OF PUSH-UPS

DATE	TIME	NUMBER OF PUSH-UPS

DATE	TIME	NUMBER OF PUSH-UPS

DATE	TIME	NUMBER OF PUSH-UPS
DATE	TIME	NUMBER OF PUSH-UPS

DATE	TIME	NUMBER OF PUSH-UPS

DATE	TIME	NUMBER OF PUSH-UPS

DATE	TIME	NUMBER OF PUSH-UPS
DATE	TIME	NUMBER OF PUSH-UPS

DATE	TIME	NUMBER OF PUSH-UPS
DATE	TIME	NUMBER OF PUSH-UPS

DATE	TIME	NUMBER OF PUSH-UPS

DATE	TIME	NUMBER OF PUSH-UPS
DATE	TIME	NUMBER OF PUSH-UPS

DATE	TIME	NUMBER OF PUSH-UPS

DATE	TIME	NUMBER OF PUSH-UPS

DATE	TIME	NUMBER OF PUSH-UPS

DATE	TIME	NUMBER OF PUSH-UPS

DATE	TIME	NUMBER OF PUSH-UPS

DATE	TIME	NUMBER OF PUSH-UPS

DATE	TIME	NUMBER OF PUSH-UPS

DATE	TIME	NUMBER OF PUSH-UPS
		NUMBER OF PUSH-UPS

DATE	TIME	NUMBER OF PUSH-UPS

DATE	TIME	NUMBER OF PUSH-UPS

DATE	TIME	NUMBER OF PUSH-UPS

DATE	TIME	NUMBER OF PUSH-UPS

DATE	TIME	NUMBER OF PUSH-UPS
DATE	TIME	NUMBER OF PUSH-UPS

DATE	TIME	NUMBER OF PUSH-UPS

DATE	TIME	NUMBER OF PUSH-UPS

DATE	TIME	NUMBER OF PUSH-UPS

DATE	TIME	NUMBER OF PUSH-UPS

DATE	TIME	NUMBER OF PUSH-UPS

DATE	TIME	NUMBER OF PUSH-UPS
DATE	TIME	NUMBER OF PUSH-UPS

DATE	TIME	NUMBER OF PUSH-UPS

DATE	TIME	NUMBER OF PUSH-UPS

DATE	TIME	NUMBER OF PUSH-UPS

DATE	TIME	NUMBER OF PUSH-UPS

DATE	TIME	NUMBER OF PUSH-UPS

DATE	TIME	NUMBER OF PUSH-UPS
DATE	TIME	NUMBER OF PUSH-UPS

DATE	TIME	NUMBER OF PUSH-UPS

DATE	TIME	NUMBER OF PUSH-UPS

DATE	TIME	NUMBER OF PUSH-UPS

DATE	TIME	NUMBER OF PUSH-UPS